FEMALE INFERTILITY

CAUSES AND NATURAL REMEDIES

ANTHONY EKANEM

Contents

Preface

Far too many women struggle to get pregnant and conceive a child naturally. This generally drives most people to visit a doctor or specialist to find out why they have so much difficulty conceiving and giving birth to healthy, happy babies. In most cases, they're given a diagnosis of infertility.

Unfortunately, there are many different reasons for infertility, so this doesn't always help. It's known that ovarian cysts, Polycystic Ovarian Syndrome (PCOS) and endometriosis can affect your fertility rate, as can a low sperm count in men. Some people are affected by other hormonal issues or more complicated problems, such as blocked or obstructed fallopian tubes.

Even with all the advances made by medical science, there remains a possibility that doctors simply can't find a cause for some peoples' infertility problems. Yet, what most people forget is that traditional, natural remedies often have a far greater success rate than expensive, often painful medical treatments.

Despite a higher success rate, many women still choose to ignore natural treatments and solutions that really could prepare their bodies to conceive naturally, even after being told that they are infertile by a medical specialist.

It's been proven that some fertility treatments prescribed by fertility specialists can increase the risk of contracting ovarian cancer, yet women every day still opt to take expensive medications rather than consider some of the healthier options of trying a holistic approach.

What's more, many of the medical treatments, surgeries and pharmaceutical drugs for infertility don't treat the base cause of the problem. Instead, they treat the symptom and attempt to remove it that way. This can sometimes cause more problems than you started with.

This Book will look at some reasons for infertility and how using a natural, holistic approach to reversing your infertility problems can greatly improve your chances of conceiving a child of your own without surgery or drugs.

So, are you ready to change your life and become a happy mother? If yes, please read on!

CHAPTER ONE

Understanding Fertility and Infertility

To achieve your goal to get pregnant fast and naturally, you need to have a deeper understanding of what fertility and infertility are all about. Only when you can recognise what your body is telling you, will you be able to address the problem and choose the perfect solution. The following paragraphs will discuss the definitions of fertility and infertility as well as their signs and causes.

What Is Female Fertility?

Female fertility is the ability of a woman to conceive and bear children. In other words, it is a woman's ability to become pregnant as a result of normal sexual activity with a man. Women generally start to become fertile between the ages of 10 and 16 when they start to go through puberty and begin menstruating. Naturally, once a woman starts her menstrual cycle, she can become pregnant if she engages in unprotected sexual activity. Cycles can be irregular for the first couple of years and many girls do not ovulate every month.

A woman's fertility will hit its peak at the age of 27 and slowly declines at the age of 30 and every year after that. That is why many older women have trouble getting pregnant. During the peak of fertility, a woman is only fertile for three to four days every cycle. This is because an unfertilized egg can only survive for 24 hours.

Signs Of Female Fertility

You can find out for yourself if you are fertile and can conceive a baby. Here are the basic signs that should tell you your fertility status:

1. Basal Body Temperature (BBT)

BBT is your body's temperature before doing any activity for the day. This is taken in the morning before you get out of bed. Your BBT when you are fertile is slightly higher than your normal temperature before your cycle. It will usually rise between 0.4 and 0.8 F on the day of ovulation.

2. Cervical Fluid

Your cervical mucus or vaginal discharge varies throughout the month and the mucus is an indicator of fertility. When you check your mucus, note the colour changes. You are at a "high fertile stage" when your mucus is thin and transparent. It has stretchy properties, and this type of mucus is also called "egg white cervical mucus".

3. Cervical Position

During your cycle, your cervix changes position. During the beginning of your cycle and after ovulation, your cervix is in a low position. It rises to a higher position just before and during the ovulation period.

What Is Female Infertility?

Contrary to fertility, female infertility is the inability of a woman to conceive and bear children during her reproductive years. Many women may be infertile during their reproductive years for various reasons. They may not be aware of the condition at the time because they were not yet seeking to have any children.

Causes Of Female Infertility

Millions of women worldwide are having fertility problems. A woman might feel or have a hunch that she could be infertile when she has not gotten pregnant after six months to one year of unprotected sex. Even a miscarriage can be an indicator of infertility. A miscarriage is a failed pregnancy experienced by women whose growing foetus was not able to complete its nine-month development stages in the womb and eventually dies. If a woman had an episode of a miscarriage, she is a likely suspect of infertility.

There are several major causes of infertility in women and knowing these causes will give you an edge in terms of deciding the right methods of treatment should you decide to get any. Here is a list of some of the major causes of infertility in women that you should know about:

1. **Polycystic Ovarian Syndrome (PCOS)**

PCOS is one of the main causes of infertility in women. This disease occurs when cysts develop in the woman's ovaries making it unable to function. When a woman has PCOS, she will experience an irregular menstrual cycle and therefore increases the probability of becoming infertile. This condition is even more depressing to bear since there is no known cure for it because doctors could not identify its causes.

2. Uterine fibroids

Upon reaching the age of 30 and above, you are at a greater risk of the development of fibroid tumours in the uterine. While these tumours are mostly benign, they can block your fallopian tubes and consequently make you infertile.

3. Ovulation disorders

One of the most recognized culprits of infertility in women is a disorder in the process of ovulation. Ovulation takes place when the ovary releases an egg down to the fallopian tube where it will become fertilized when it meets a sperm. But there are a few cases where a certain part of the brain responsible for ovulation is disrupted and decreasing the levels of important hormones in the process. These hormones aid ovulation. This small yet caustic abnormality prevents the ovary from releasing the egg.

4. Endometriosis

A problem in the lining of the uterus can also be a cause of infertility in women. This condition cuts down your chances of getting pregnant as uterine tissue grows outside of the uterus and oftentimes affects the ovaries, uterus, and fallopian tubes. This growth is also known as an endometrial cyst which is common in the ovary and can either be benign or malignant.

5. Age

A woman's rich reproductive age is in her early and mid-twenties and starts to decline in her late twenties and every year after reaching the age of thirty. Fertility declines rapidly as we age, especially in women, because our general health also declines.

6. Fallopian Tube Blockages

Blocked or damaged fallopian tubes are thought to account for up to 40% of female infertility problems. Blocked tubes will prevent eggs from reaching the uterus and prevent sperm from reaching the egg. In most cases, women have no idea their tubes might be blocked, as there are generally no obvious symptoms to look for.

There are two types of blocked tubes – partial blockage and Hydro-salpinx. A partial blockage may be a result of endometrial lining closing off a portion of the tube, which can result in a tubal pregnancy or ectopic pregnancy. A hydro-salpinx is when the tube is completely blocked and begins to fill with fluid, which makes the tube dilate and swell as it fills. If both tubes are affected, the chances of conceiving are zero.

The predominant causes of blocked tubes are a history of Pelvic Inflammatory Disease, Chlamydia, ruptured appendix, endometriosis, or other types of uterine infection.

Infertility specialists will advise that laparoscopic surgery is required to unblock the affected tubes. However, this can cause further scarring in some cases. In the case of a hydro-salpinx, a specialist may advise that a hydro-salpingectomy is required, which is a complete removal of the dilated fallopian tube. This destroys any chance of getting pregnant naturally in future and the patient becomes dependent on IVF treatments if further children are wanted.

Once again, there are plenty of non-surgical options available to help unblock damaged fallopian tubes. Alternative therapies that include manual physical therapy have also shown positive results.

CHAPTER TWO

Starting a Family

Starting your family is one of the most exciting times of your life. Having a child ranks as one of the most life-changing and rewarding decisions you will ever make.

For some lucky couples, the road to parenthood is smooth and short. Unfortunately, a lot of couples find the road is filled with anxiety and stress as they discover that getting pregnant is more difficult and takes longer than they originally thought. Hopefully, this book will equip you with the knowledge you need to make your journey to parenthood worry-free and successful.

You Are Not Alone

Whether you have just started or have been trying to get pregnant for a while, be patient. It sometimes takes time to conceive. Getting pregnant is not like flipping on a switch.

When everything is done right and there are no complications, the average healthy couple has a 25% chance of getting pregnant each month. So, if you have been trying for four months or more, don't give up hope. You are not alone. There are millions of couples who are trying to conceive at any given moment with similar success rates. Most likely, it is just the luck of the draw.

Luckily, there are things you can do to increase your odds each month. This guide will give you the knowledge you need to enhance your efforts and make sure you have the best possible chance each month.

Should You Be Concerned with Infertility?

A diagnosis of infertility is given to couples who have been trying to conceive for 12 months or more without success. Most health care professionals believe you should be able to conceive within a year. If you have been trying for 12 months or longer without success, it is time to contact your obstetrician or a fertility specialist and have a fertility evaluation.

It is important that both partners are examined because fertility issues could be attributed to either one of you – or both. About one-third of all infertility cases are accounted for by the woman's reproductive health, one third by the man's reproductive health, and one-third collectively as a couple. Any recommendations for continuing the journey to conceive or how you grow your family will depend on the results of the examination.

Starting The Journey

More than likely, you are just getting started and want to do things right. This guide will provide you with all the right steps. To begin, we will explore the basics of ovulation—the foundation to conceiving— followed by ways to track your monthly ovulation cycle.

This guide will also identify nutritional and health tips for both men and women to enhance fertility. We will also make sure you are doing things right in the bedroom while keeping it fun.

Congratulations – growing your family is a time for fun and celebration. Delivering a "big fat positive" on your pregnancy test is our goal, and this guide will maximize your efforts and give you the knowledge you need to achieve that success.

CHAPTER THREE

Ovulation: The Key to Conception

Understanding Ovulation is the key to conception. The bottom line is that all couples want to know when the best time is to have sex to get pregnant. From the egg's perspective, there is only a 12-to-24-hour period where a woman can conceive. So how do you know when your window of conception is? The answer lies around ovulation. By understanding your ovulation cycle, you can target the optimal time frame for conception.

Some of the most common questions about ovulation are:

- When does ovulation occur—before or after my period?
- Is it best to have sex before or during ovulation?
- What day of the month gives me the greatest chance of conception?

Those are important questions. To answer them, we need to learn the basics of ovulation.

Ovulation Basics

To begin, let's nail down what we mean by ovulation. Ovulation is the point when an egg is released from the ovary so that it may travel down the fallopian tube and become fertilized by a waiting sperm. During ovulation, the lining of the uterine wall thickens so that a fertilized egg can become implanted and continue the pregnancy.

Essential Ovulation Facts

- An egg is only available for fertilization for 12 to 24 hours
- Usually, only 1 egg is released during each cycle
- Ovulation often rotates between ovaries
- Light bleeding may occur during ovulation
- It is possible to ovulate even if a period has not occurred

Before Or After My Period?

Does ovulation occur before or after my period? This is one of the most common questions asked by women beginning to track their ovulation. Technically, ovulation *should* occur around 14 days before your period. However, in terms of tracking your ovulation, it may be better to think of it occurring in the middle, about halfway between two periods for an average 28-day cycle.

Let's assume you have a 28-day cycle each month. If you count 14 days backwards from the first day of any period (the day bleeding starts), or if you count 14 days forwards from the first day of any period, you will find that ovulation should occur on day 14 or 15 of your cycle — either way you count. Because 14, the average day of ovulation, is exactly half of a 28-day cycle, it is mathematically in the middle.

The problem is no one is average—every woman is different. Your cycles could be 32 days on average and not 28. On top of that, cycles are not always the same length each month. One month may be longer than the next. History does not always predict the future. As we will see, there is only a small chance ovulation will occur on day 14 of your cycle.

The 14 Day Fallacy

Most clinical guidelines, doctors and reproductive professionals still state with absolute certainty that ovulation occurs exactly 14 days before your period regardless of the woman or her cycle. As we know from recent studies, that belief is just wrong. The data shows that ovulation rarely occurs 14 days before a woman's next period.

A study by Allen J. Wilcox of the National Institute of Environmental Health Sciences tracked ovulations in 696 menstrual cycles and found that *"...only a small percentage of women ovulate exactly 14 days before the onset of [her period]. This is true even for women whose cycles are usually 28 days long. Among the 696 cycles for 28 days in our study, ovulation occurred 14 days before the next [period] in only 10%. Time from ovulation to next menses ranged from 7 to 19 days (days 10 to 22 of the menstrual cycle)."*

Many couples could be missing critical opportunities for conception each month. For some, the added stress and frustration of months of unsuccessful attempts could be due in part to this false 14-day rule.

So how do you know when ovulation occurs? The bottom line is that you can't predict with certainty the day ovulation will occur in each month, going strictly by when your last period started. Remember, your last period was triggered by the timing of your last ovulation and has no relation to the next ovulation. You could be early or late this month. But on average, ovulation should occur around day 14 or 15 for most women with a 28-day cycle. Notice we said, *on average, should,* and *around.* We just can't rely on what *should* happen as gospel. Remember the Wilcox study showed it ranged from 7 to 19 days before the next period — and that is just for women with regular 28-day cycles.

Fertile Window

*When should you time sex for the best chance of getting pregnant?*Again, it all relates to your ovulation. Let's pretend for a moment we *can* pinpoint when ovulation will occur. According to statistical data, there are exactly 6 days each cycle where you have a chance of conceiving (we know we said the egg was only available for 12 to 24 hours, we will explain the difference later). They include the day of ovulation and the 5 days just before ovulation. Outside of this window, your chances drop to near zero. The two days before ovulation presents the best chance of all, followed by the day before and the day of ovulation. This critical six-day window is commonly referred to as your fertile window. Knowing when this six-day window occurs in your cycle is important to increase your chance of getting pregnant.

*If predicting your day of ovulation is impossible, how are you supposed to know when your fertile window is?*While it is true that predicting the exact day of your ovulation, and therefore your fertile window, is impossible by estimating your last period—we do have some good guesses when it will occur on average. At least that is a start.

When it comes to traditional clinical guidelines, most state that an average woman with a 28-day cycle will experience her fertile window between day 10 and day 17 of her cycle (day 1 being the first day of her last period). This information is wrong on two fronts! So, let's look at correcting it to fit the actual data.

First, the clinical guidelines assume that the fertile windows include the 5 days before ovulation, the day of ovulation and two days after ovulation. We know from several studies that the chance of pregnancy occurring after the day of ovulating drops drastically to below 5% with most calculating it at closer to 0% than 5%. The second issue is that more than 10% of women are already in their fertile window by day 7 of their cycle!

Since your day of ovulation varies month to month, your 6-day fertile window varies and is just as hard to predict based on your last period. A much better approach is to look at all the days of the month and see, based on statistical data, what the probability is of being in your 6-day fertile window for each day. To say it differently, what are all the days during your cycle when there is a chance you are in your fertile window and therefore can get pregnant. Fortunately, that is just what the 2000 Wilcox study was looking for.

The Fertile Phase of Your Cycle

Before we look more closely at the Wilcox study, let's better define what we are looking for. We'll call it the fertile phase (not to be confused with the *fertile window*). The fertile phase of your cycle expands the fertile window (those 6 days of the month where intercourse can result in pregnancy) to include all the days in your cycle in which you *may be* within the window. That is the fertile phase that incudes any day in your cycle where sexual intercourse could result in pregnancy.

To define the fertile phase of your cycle, we also need to define a cut-off in terms of the probability of getting pregnant. It would be impractical to say your fertile phase includes all days with a probability greater than 0% of getting pregnant. Likewise, we don't want to miss any opportunity for conception by setting the cut-off too high – say 15% or more.

Turns out that setting the cut-off to include all days with a greater than 5% chance should cover our bases just fine.

We know from the Wilcox study and other statistical research that most women have a 5% or greater chance of being in their fertile window anywhere from day 6 to day 21 of their cycle. Therefore, the fertile phase for most women occurs during those 16 days between day 6 and day 21 of the cycle.

The internet is loaded with articles that still repeat the old clinical guidelines recommending couples focus conception efforts only on days 10 to 17 — the traditional definition of the fertile window. If you follow those guidelines, you are missing the boat on opportunities for conception.

Instead, you should focus your efforts on the fertile phase of your cycle between days 7 and day 20 (or between day 6 and day 21 if you want a little extra insurance). However, if you have a history of irregular cycles, your fertile phase can be much longer. You must learn to recognize your *signs of ovulation* so at least you know when ovulation has occurred, and conception opportunities are over for that
month.

Signs Of Ovulation

Ovulation varies from woman to woman and even cycle to cycle. However, the biological changes that occur during ovulation are fairly consistent for each person. There are primary symptoms that should be experienced by all women, and you should be able to readily spot them.

Primary Symptoms of Ovulation:

- Change in cervical mucus becoming more slippery
- Spike in basal body temperatures

- •Change in cervical position or firmness

There are additional signs of ovulation that may not be experienced by all women and may take some effort in recognizing.

Secondary Symptoms of Ovulation:

- Light spotting
- Cramping
- Pain on one side
- Bloating
- Breast tenderness
- Increased libido
- Heightened sense of smell, taste or even vision

You may not notice any of these secondary symptoms of your ovulation, and that is fine. If you do notice, then these signs can help you track your ovulation. Some women are good enough at recognizing their symptoms that they can tell soon enough in advance of ovulation when to target their sexual encounters for that critical sweet spot in the fertile window two days before ovulation.

It is important to know that tracking your ovulation is not impossible. In the next chapter, we will gain more insight on predicting the critical 6-day fertile window with more accuracy. For most though, it will just come down to having sex the right number of times during the right phase of the month to cover your bases. That, of course, is the easiest, no-cost, fool-proof way to get pregnant.

CHAPTER FOUR

Tracking Your Ovulation

Knowing when your ovulation occurs makes it easy for couples to target when to have sex. However, we found out in the last chapter that tracking your ovulation based on your last period is problematic. Don't worry; there are other more reliable ways to track your ovulation. But be careful. Tracking ovulation can easily become clinical and makes sex more of a chore if you are not protective of the relationship and only focused on the job of getting pregnant. It is important to keep the romance and spontaneity in a relationship.

Key Facts

As noted in the last chapter, the egg is available for fertilization for only 12 to 24 hours a cycle. This is a very short time frame! You would think that would make it extremely difficult in timing intercourse for conception.

Didn't you say the fertile window was six days and not 24 hours? The 12 to 24 hours is just when the *egg* is available for conception. Unlike the egg, sperm is available any time. More importantly, sperm can live inside the uterus for 2, 3 and even up to 5 days. This is part of the reason the fertile window is 6 days and not 12 to 24 hours.

Additionally, conception is more likely if the sperm is waiting for the egg. Therefore, it is best to have sperm waiting inside for the egg versus trying to have sex at the point of ovulation. This leeway gives you much more flexibility than trying to precisely time
ovulation.

So how can we track ovulation? There are two basic approaches to tracking ovulation. One approach uses a calendar and a guess at when ovulation should occur, or better yet when it is possible to get pregnant during a cycle. The other approach measures physical changes in the body to determine ovulation. Better techniques can pinpoint the important two days before ovulation when you have the greatest chance of conceiving.

The Calendar Methods

There are several calendar-based methods for targeting ovulation and timing intercourse for conception. They go by different names – the Rhythm Method, Standard Days Method, etc. Some are complicated and require you to track your periods for several months and make calculations. Others ask you to note the first day of your period and then count out a certain number of days to target sex for that month. Unfortunately, most are based on the same flawed assumptions we pointed out in the last chapter. If you have been using these methods, you could be missing key opportunities for conception each month. Let's look at a couple.

Simple Calendar Method

One of the simplest calendar methods requires you to simply count out 10 days from the first day of your period (day 1 is the first day you bleed). Then, have sex every other day until day 21. This is using the 6-day "fertility window" discussed in the previous chapter with some wiggle room to account for variances in your ovulation from month to month.

But this method assumes that ovulation won't start sooner than day 14 of the cycle. We know from the Wilcox study that 10% of women are already in their fertile window by day 7. Also, women with irregular cycles could ovulate much later than day 21.

As added evidence, just look at the high failure rates of calendar methods like the one above when they are used to avoid pregnancy. For couples using these methods as a form of birth control, the estimated failure rates are over 25% per year. That equates to one in four couples who use a traditional calendar method that end up pregnant when they were not supposed to.

Conversely, it stands to reason the opposite holds true - out of all the couples using a traditional calendar method to try and conceive, a significant percentage are missing their fertile window each month.

Standard Days Method

To counter the high failure rates in traditional calendar approaches, a new method was developed in 1999 by Georgetown University's Institute for Reproductive Health called the standards day method. It uses the concept of the fertile phase we introduced in the last chapter.

Consequently, this method divides a woman's cycle into three phases:

1. **Menstruation Infertile: Day 1-7.**
   This phase is during your period and immediately afterwards where it is assumed no egg is present for fertilization.

2. **Fertile: Day 8-19.** This time frame assumes ovulation occurs around day 15 and that conception can occur up to four days after ovulation (which is false).

3. **Infertile:** From Day 20, infertility is assumed to resume. However, women with irregular or longer cycles could still be in their fertility window.

Though this method uses some of the same flawed assumptions that the other calendar methods use, it is easy to understand and has a much lower failure rate when used for pregnancy prevention. Unfortunately, it is still missing critical days on each end of the fertile phase. Remember, the Wilcox study clearly shows that between days 6 and 21 of the cycle, women had a greater than 10% probability of being in their fertile window.

Modified Standard Days Method

Because the Wilcox study mentioned in the last chapter was published after the Standard Days Method was developed in 1999, it was not yet clear that the fertile phase could start as early as day 6 or last longer than day 19. This new data suggests the Standard Days Method needs some updating. When it comes to trying to conceive, you don't want to leave any opportunity on the table.

Therefore, the *American Pregnancy Association* recommends couples use a Modified Standards Days method of targeting fertility with a 14-day fertile phase.

- Menstruation Infertile: Day 1-6
- Fertile: Day 7-20
- Infertile: From Day 21.

Want to get pregnant the quickest and easiest way possible without using messy test strips or expensive monitors? Use the modified standards days method and commit to having sex 4 to 7 times during your 14-day fertile phase. You'll greatly increase your chances without the stress and complications of other methods.

Create a schedule!

Do yourself a favour and start using this modified calendar approach today to help you conceive:

1. On the first day of your period (the first day you notice bleeding) mark your calendar. This is Day 1 of your cycle.

2. Count forward 6 more days. This is day 7 of your cycle. This is the start of your Fertile Phase.

3. Mark or colour in your 14-day fertile phase including all the days between day 7and day 20 of your cycle (include both day 7 and day 20). If you want, you can add day 6 and day 21 for extra assurance.

Now let the fun begin with a focus on sex every other day. The reason you want to have sex every other day is to maximize the health of your partner's sperm. Too much sex can result in immature sperm and long bouts without sex can lead to ejaculating fluid with dead or weakened sperm. With sperm living 2, 3 and even up to 5 days, sex every other day gives you plenty of sperm for conception to occur.

Keep in mind, this method is most reliable for women with cycles shorter than 32 days. Women with long cycles or who are highly irregular will need to track ovulation more closely.

However, for the average couple, this method is the best and easiest way of targeting ovulation and maximizing your efforts for getting pregnant. If you want, you can augment this calendar method with the fertility awareness techniques we will explain in the next section.

Fertility Awareness and Ovulation Monitoring

Pinpointing your actual day of ovulation, or more important, knowing when you enter your peak, 6-day fertile window can increase your chances of getting pregnant. Studies show that timing sex to occur exactly 2 days before your ovulation day results in the greatest chance of pregnancy.

So, by knowing the onset of ovulation, you can increase your odds of success. If you follow our advice of sex every other day during the 14 days of your "fertile phase," you will have covered your bases without the need for the extra work. But for some couples, this added information can help by focusing their efforts around 6 days of their fertile window instead of the full 14 days of the fertile phase.

Furthermore, it is important for women with cycles greater than 32 days or irregular cycles to track their ovulation more accurately. Ovulation can occur much later than day 20 for long or irregular cycles

The Modified Standards Day method we outlined previously is not designed for use for women with cycles longer than 32 days or irregular cycles. If you use this method, you could be missing your fertility window altogether. This is where fertility awareness and ovulation monitoring come in.

Fertility Awareness

Fertility Awareness (sometimes called natural family planning) involves monitoring temperatures with a basal thermometer and checking the *cervical mucus* to pinpoint your actual day of ovulation. Right before ovulation, the cervical mucus becomes wet and slippery and will remain this way until the ovulation process has been completed. Some people describe the texture as like "egg whites." It becomes stretchier and more elastic-like between your fingers if you press them together and pull them apart.

In addition to monitoring cervical mucus, a *basal thermometer* is used to track your temperature. It is extremely sensitive and will reflect a spike in your temperature that happens when ovulation occurs. There are fertility charts that you can use to record the temperatures and make it easier to notice the shifts in temperature.

Fertility Awareness is a great way to become in touch with your body. Some women get to know their cycles so well that they can know when ovulation is pending or happening by the way their bodies change. However, fertility awareness does take practice and most people find it helpful to go to a fertility awareness or natural family planning class to make sure they are fully trained.

Ovulation Tests and Monitors

Many women and couples have busy schedules which create challenges for trying to employ the 14-day calendar method or the detailed fertility awareness method. This is one of the reasons that some women and couples turn to ovulation tests and monitors.

Ovulation tests involve a series of test strips that you use to detect the luteinizing hormone (LH) surge in your urine just before you ovulate. The benefit of ovulation test strips is that the surge in LH occurs in that critical 3-day window before ovulation. Remember, this is the timeframe with the greatest chance of conception. Therefore, ovulation test strips make it much easier to time sex in the important 3-2 days before ovulation when you have your greatest chances for success.

To use the strips, calculate the basic window of anticipated ovulation and then begin testing with a strip each morning. Once the tests turn back positive, you have identified your ovulation. But be careful. Testing with the first morning urine can cause false positives. Most test kits recommend testing twice a day between 10 AM and 8 PM. In addition to ovulation tests, there are several different types of fertility monitors on the market. They typically work by having you input the first day of your period and then they track one or more hormones to calculate your two peak fertile days as well as your 6-day fertile window.

In addition to monitors, there is also a fertility watch that works a little differently. You simply wear it to bed each night and it will give you advance notice of when your 6-day fertile window is. Once in the window, it will indicate what day of the window you are in. Many women like the watch because they don't have to worry about using messy urine test strips.

Subtle Signs of Ovulation

Whichever method you employ, it helps to be in tune with your body to recognize the signs of ovulation yourself. The more you pay attention to your body and your cycle, the greater chance you will have of keying into these signs of ovulation.

- Light spotting
- Cramping
- Pain on one side
- Bloating
- Breast tenderness
- Increased libido
- Heightened sense of smell, taste or even vision

Don't worry if you are not noticing these symptoms, it is common not to. But if you are recognizing them month to month, then you can add these into your ovulation tracking practices making your conception efforts more purposeful and accurate.

Making The Choice

The calendar method, fertility awareness, or ovulation testing are all viable ways to help you learn about your cycle and identify when ovulation occurs each month. The important thing is for you to begin to understand your body and your cycle. A well-informed woman is more likely to conceive without the happenstance shots in the dark.

For women with regular 28–32-day cycles

For the average couple where the woman experiences regular cycles between 28 and32 days, the most effective and easiest way to get pregnant is the Modified Standard Days calendar method. If you have the freedom to enjoy the bedroom every other day during the 14-day fertile phase of your cycle, then this method is the route you should go. If you can't do it every other day, then shoot for every three days which will still leave you with a great chance of conceiving.

The Modified Standard Days method is absolutely the best way to get pregnant and there is no need to invest in expensive monitors or worry with test strips if you don't want to. But if you want, you can complement this route with either the fertility awareness approach or the testing/ monitor route to help pinpoint your peak fertile day 2 days before your ovulation when you have the greatest chance of getting pregnant.

Women with irregular/long cycles, or older couples

Unfortunately, the Modified Standard Days method is only designed to work for women with fairly standard, regular cycles between 28 and 32 days. If your cycles are longer or irregular, you need to invest in tracking your ovulation more closely. For those that fall into this category, we highly recommend you learn to recognize your secondary signs of ovulation and invest in test strips, a basal thermometer, or a fertility monitor. A monitor that accurately pinpoints your fertile window along with the peak fertile day 2 days before ovulation is the best route to go.

We also recommend couples 35 and older invest in a fertility monitor. Older couples have lower chances of conceiving each month versus those under the age of 35. In addition, older women are more prone to ovulation failure and tend to have shorter cycles. Fertility tracking with a monitor or fertility awareness will give you the boost you need to overcome these additional challenges

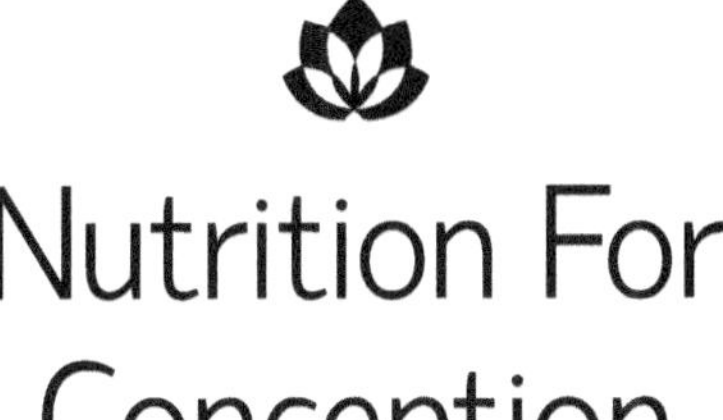

Nutrition For Conception

Women and couples who are trying to conceive often look for the inside scoop on what they can do to maximize their chances. One of the questions often asked is, *"Are there any foods I can eat to help me conceive?"* The answer is yes, but up until recently, there has been little research on the influence of diets on fertility. As research emerges, we are getting a better picture of how diet and specific foods can affect fertility – especially when it comes to what *not* to eat. Be careful, there are still a lot of myths, misconceptions and wrong advice floating around. We'll try and stick to just the facts.

Nutrition For Conception

One of the best ways to invest in your chances for conception is to be healthy yourself. One thing we do know is a healthy body increases your chances of conception and enhances the health and wellness of your baby.

You are what you eat. Eating healthy and well-balanced meals helps your body to work to the best of its ability. The objective is to consume the recommended amounts of carbohydrates, fibre, protein, essential fats, and water daily.

Hopefully, you have been practising healthy eating throughout your life. But if not, you should give yourself at least three months of healthy nutrition before trying to conceive. That goes for both of you.

Healthy nutrition is linked to fertility for both men and women. Therefore, you both must eat well-balanced meals. It is an investment in both you and your fertility. Research is affirming what nutritionists believed – our body reacts negatively to the junk that gets put into it and works better when given what it needs.

Foods To Avoid

Caffeine: Caffeine is not good for your baby, but research is also showing that it can lower your fertility by approximately 27%. Caffeine also has a negative effect on your overall nutrition because it restricts the body's ability to absorb iron and calcium.

Processed Foods: Highly processed foods contribute to obesity and can contain pesticides, artificial hormones, and preservatives. These foods negatively affect your fertility by decreasing your hormonal health. Instead, try and eat organic and choose foods that you recognize as coming from a farm as opposed to a factory. Avoid the cookies, chips, boxed convenience items and frozen meals in favour of fresh fruits, vegetables, meat, and dairy. A good rule of thumb is to avoid any packaged item with more than five ingredients.

Red Meat: Diets that are high in red meat consumption are tied to health concerns that can impact your fertility such as endometriosis. Yes, red meat is indeed a good source of iron which is an important mineral for conception health. However, recent studies show the type of Iron in plant-based sources to be more effective in conception health and preventing ovulation failure. There have been no such links established for animal-based sources of iron as found in red meat. Therefore, it is best to limit red meat consumption while trying to conceive.

Soy Products: Soy-based products have been shown to decrease sperm counts in men in several studies. It appears that an *isoflavone* compound called *Genistein,* found in all soy-containing products, slows, or even destroys human sperm. Men should avoid products like soy milk, tofu, edamame, and other soybean-based products – at least while you are trying to conceive.

For women, soybeans can be an excellent source of plant-based protein, contain a natural form of estrogen and have many positive health attributes. However, the jury is still out on their overall effect on women's fertility. Studies have shown that even small amounts of the compound *Genistein* in the female tract could destroy sperm. Therefore, even women should avoid soy products—at least during ovulation and limit their amounts during other times of the month.

Refined Sugars and Simple Carbohydrates: You should *avoid* eating simple carbohydrates that include sugar, white pasta, white flour, other refined grains and unfortunately sweets. One of the reasons to avoid these simple carbohydrates is because they cause your body to use up more nutrients to process than they provide – a net loss for you and your fertility. However, the biggest reason is their implication in overall weight gain and our obesity epidemic. It is a fact—overweight couples are less fertile.

Bad Fats: When it comes to health in general, there are good fats and there are bad fats. Research increasingly points to links with bad fats like the trans fats (partially hydrogenated fats) found in processed foods and the saturated fats in animal meat with lower fertility rates.

Therefore, trans fats and saturated fats should be eliminated from your diet and replaced with good fats like mono-unsaturated fat found in olive oil.

Fertility Diet Basics

You now know that healthy nutrition directly relates to healthy fertility, and you know what kinds of foods to avoid. Let's take it to the next level and talk about key factors of a nutritional plan targeted towards conception.

Water: Drink lots of water! Water is important for organ function by serving as the mechanism for helping to deliver nutrients to your body. It also influences your hormonal balance, and we all know the importance of hormones and pregnancy. Furthermore, water cleanses and helps carry toxins out of your body allowing it to function at optimal levels and helps prevent those toxins from building up and negatively impacting your fertility.

Complex Carbohydrates: Eating complex carbohydrates like vegetables, whole grains, brown rice, and whole-grain cereals and pasta are some of the best ways to get the nutrients that positively influence your fertility. Although fruits are simple carbohydrates, you should still include them in your dietary intake because they include other nutrients that are favourable for conception.

The complex carbohydrates of vegetables, whole grains and fruits also ensure that you have fibre in your diet. Along with water, fibre works to help remove toxins from your system keeping your organs and body in healthy working condition.

Protein: Protein influences your fertility by providing the nutrients that contribute towards hormone production. Some protein should be consumed during every meal; however, it is important what type of protein you eat. Diets that are high in red meat consumption are tied to health concerns that can impact your fertility such as endometriosis. The best proteins come from eggs, beans, nuts, seeds, oily fish, and white meat. If you must eat red meat, choose lean cuts, and avoid processed meats like bacon and sausage. Also, make sure you avoid fish that are high in mercury.

Good Fats: There are different types of fats, and they are important to your fertility. The fatty acids found in oily fish, nuts and seeds affect both fertility and the healthy development of your growing baby during pregnancy. The trans fats in processed foods and the saturated fats in animal meat are the ones that can have a negative impact on your fertility and should be avoided.

Essential fatty acids can be obtained in oily fish like mackerel and salmon, as well as nuts and seeds. You can also complement your food intake with Omega-3 fish oil supplements. The FDA recommends that women eat up to 12 ounces a week of fish that are low in mercury to get the Omega-3 fatty acids needed for healthy fertility and baby development.

Whole Milk: Although it is best to avoid saturated fats, especially from animal sources, there is new research around milk fat. Studies have pointed to a link between drinking whole milk and increased fertility rates in women. Researchers found that women who drank 3 or more glasses of whole milk a day were 70% less likely to be infertile due to failed ovulation.

It appears the natural hormones found in whole milk fat seem to give a boost to fertility in women. If the milk fat is removed, the natural hormones left in non-fat milk seem to decrease fertility in women by increasing ovulation failure rates. Therefore, it is recommended that women switch to limited amounts of whole milk while trying to conceive.

Try replacing the milk in your morning cereal with whole milk. For dessert at night, try whole-milk ice cream instead. If you are not a milk drinker, try whole-milk yoghurt for a snack. It is important you talk with your doctor first if you have high cholesterol or a history of heart disease. Remember, whole milk is high in saturated fat which could compound those conditions and should be avoided normally. So only switch to whole milk during the months you are trying to conceive and limit the amount of whole milk. The study shows that as little as one 8oz serving of whole milk can significantly increase fertility rates.

Essential Nutrients for Her

There are no magical nutrients that will get you pregnant. If there were, we would be the first in line to market the pills! Any fertility diet is first off grounded in sound nutritional eating for overall good health. A healthy diet will impact the fertility of both you and your partner. With that said, some key nutrients directly affect fertility in women:

Zinc: Zinc directly impacts fertility in women. There is plenty of research tying deficiencies in zinc with negative effects on fertility for both men and women. Accordingly, men and women should keep the dietary allowance of 15mg of zinc daily as part of their regular food intake. Getting zinc naturally can be done by eating vegetables, eggs, whole grains, nuts, sunflower seeds, watermelon, and dried fruit. You can also find zinc in onions, beetroot, peas, and beans.

Vitamin B6: Vitamin B6 affects your fertility by contributing to the production of female sex hormones and by regulating both estrogen and progesterone. B6 increases your chances of conception and decreases your chances of miscarriage. Getting B6 naturally can be done so by eating eggs, salmon, peanuts, bananas, soybeans, and sunflower seeds. Prenatal vitamins will also contain B6 as part of the supplement and are a great way to ensure that you have this essential fertility and baby wellness nutrient.

Vitamin C: Vitamin C is a fertility nutrient because it helps in triggering ovulation. It also helps in sperm count for men, so it plays a key role for both men and women. Vitamin C can be consumed through vegetables and fruits in particular: strawberries, oranges, kiwi, mangoes, and blueberries.

Vitamin E: Vitamin E is another fertility nutrient for both men and women, enhances hormone function in women and affects sperm function in men. Vitamin E can be obtained naturally through oily fish, green leafy vegetables, broccoli, nuts, egg yolk, whole grains, and unrefined oils.

Essential Nutrients for Him

Fertility is not just a woman's thing. More and more research is showing that healthy fertility is related to the health of both the man and the woman. Eating well-balanced meals is the starting place. Here are some key nutrients he wants to make sure he is getting.

Zinc: Zinc is an important nutrient that contributes to the production of semen and testosterone in men. It impacts both the quality and production of sperm.

Vitamin C: Vitamin C helps prevent sperm from clumping together and improves sperm count.

Vitamin E: Vitamin E also increases sperm quality - especially when combined with selenium.

Omega 3 Fatty Acids: Omega-3s enhance sperm quality and viability. All these nutrients have been tied to healthy sperm production and function. Men should make sure that they are getting their recommended daily doses.

Nutrition For Baby Wellness

Eating well-balanced meals is an investment in your body, your fertility, and your baby. It is important you start preparing for a healthy pregnancy before you conceive to ensure both healthy foetal development and to minimize or prevent pregnancy complications.

Healthy foetal development

The following nutrients may not affect your chances of conceiving, but they do invest in your baby from the get-go. You should include these vitamins and minerals in your conception diet because your baby will need them from the first days of development and throughout the pregnancy.

Folic Acid - make sure that you are getting at least 400 micrograms daily before conception. You should increase it to 800 micrograms after conception. Folic acid can be consumed through dark leafy vegetables, whole grains, fortified bread and cereals and prenatal vitamins.

Calcium - women need to get at least 1,000mgs of calcium a day. Calcium contributes to bone development. You can consume calcium through milk, cottage cheese, yoghurt, and some cheeses.

Preventing Pregnancy Complications

These nutrients should be taken as part of your fertility diet because they help prevent abnormalities in the baby during pregnancy and help decrease the chances of miscarrying.

Magnesium: Magnesium helps maintain the pregnancy. Great food sources include eggs, green vegetables, nuts, brown rice, and bananas.

Selenium: Selenium helps avoid a miscarriage and is found in eggs, whole wheat, carrots, mushrooms, tuna, and broccoli.

Manganese: Manganese helps prevent abnormalities and behaviour problems. Eggs, bananas, strawberries, apples, pineapples, onions, and legumes are great sources for manganese.

Should You Start Prenatal Vitamin Supplements Now?

Yes! You should start taking prenatal vitamins while trying to conceive. Why before? Remember that a healthy you is an investment in a healthy conception and a healthy pregnancy. By starting prenatal vitamins now, your body will already be prepared and in top shape, once you are pregnant. This will help minimize complications and ensure healthy foetal development. In addition, many of the key nutrients for conception are found in prenatal vitamins.

Checklist For Conception Nutrition

1. Eat nutritional and well-balanced meals as an investment in your body, your fertility, and your baby.

2. Focus on organic foods that include fruits, vegetables, and whole grains which also give you many of the nutrients you need for fertility wellness.

3. Remove the nutritional negatives: red meats, artificial sweeteners, simple carbohydrates, processed foods, and caffeine.

4. Get your key nutrients from natural foods first and add supplements like a pre-natal vitamin, Omega-3s, Vitamin Cs and Zinc to cover your bases.

5. Drink lots of water for good hydration, delivering the nutrients and clearing out the toxins.

6. Consider adding whole milk from sources like ice cream, whole-milk yoghurt, and whole milk on your cereal each morning.

7. Avoid consuming soybeans and other soy-based products if you're a man. Women should consider eliminating them altogether or at least in the two weeks during your ovulation window.

CHAPTER SIX

Pre-Conception Health Checklists for Women

The journey of trying to conceive can be a jungle littered with old wives' tales and myths that may or may not be true. One thing we know with certainty is that a healthy body increases the chances of conception. But there is more to health than just nutrition. This chapter covers the broader aspects of health while focusing on the known health tips and checklists that can give you an edge in getting pregnant.

Lifestyle Changes

Some key lifestyle changes are directly related to the health of your fertility and your baby. Illicit drug and alcohol abuse are harmful to your body. Any toxin you put in your body has the potential to decrease fertility rates and worse – harm the foetus after conception.

Here is a list of drugs, chemicals, and toxins you need to eliminate or quit as you are pursuing conception and the dream of a healthy baby:

- Smoking and nicotine intake
- Alcohol consumption
- Illicit drug use

- Prescription medication (consult your health care provider)
- Hazardous chemicals (work or recreation environment)
- Caffeine use

There are many things you can do which are an investment in your health and thus an investment in the health of your fertility and future baby. Here is a list of lifestyle changes that you can add to your daily routine:

- Exercise and physical activity
- Yoga
- Relaxation techniques
- Sleep and rest
- Well balanced meals
- Prenatal supplements

Nutrition And Weight

As we addressed in the previous chapter, there are some important vitamins and minerals for fertility health. Here is a list of nutrients that you need to make sure you are getting every day:

Apart from the nutritional intake, you also want to focus on your weight. Ideally, you are neither overweight nor underweight. Avoid any drastic diets to lose weight - the drastic shift can cause more harm than good. Focus on eating well and seek to incorporate smaller portions while incorporating exercise. Talk to your health care provider if you are either over or underweight about the best plan for your fertility.

Physical Health

You may be eating well and physically active only to have your fertility impaired from other health conditions.

You should get a physical check-up allowing your health care provider to evaluate:

- Diabetes or risks for gestational diabetes
- High blood pressure
- Anaemia
- Thyroid concerns
- STDs
- Blood type (Rh + or -)
- Immunity to Rubella
- Immunity to Varicella
- Pap smear for cervical dysplasia

Medical History

You should also meet with your doctor and review your medical history. A medical and family history is going to examine:

- Medications you are taking
- History with any previous pregnancies
- Physical health including dietary intake, physical activity
- Current medical conditions
- Family History
- Basic genetic screening and referrals as needed

Taking a comprehensive look at your health and making positive changes for the better is the most important step you can take in preparing for conception. You will not only be increasing your chances for a successful conception, but you'll also set the stage for a healthy, successful pregnancy. Furthermore, these checklists serve as the foundation for any fertility assessment if you end up experiencing any challenges with getting pregnant.

CHAPTER SEVEN

Having Sex for Pregnancy

Is there a right way to perform sexual intercourse to increase your chance of getting pregnant? It is not a question of whether you can get pregnant or not with different sexual positions. Conception can occur any time semen comes in contact with the vaginal area. It is more important you do things right to maximize the health of the man's sperm.

What Is the Best Position?

What is the best sexual position for getting pregnant? As noted, conception can occur with any sexual position, and studies have failed to show any significant link between sex positions and conception rates. Be careful, almost anything you hear about this topic is probably a myth or misconception.

If you have to pick one position, the "missionary" (guy on top) approach is probably the best. This starts the seminal fluid following ejaculation in the right direction from the get-go. Even better is the modified missionary position with her legs elevated up over his shoulders. This position allows for the deepest penetration and maximum gravitational aid.

Are there any bad positions? Again, pregnancy can occur with any coital position that results in sperm entering the vaginal area. But assuming we want gravity on our side, any position where the woman is on top might be inferior to others. The important thing is to spice things up and enjoy sex. Feel free to add variety to your routine, and then for extra insurance, switch back to the missionary position right before and during his orgasm.

The Gravitational Pull

Am I losing any chance of conception when the semen begins to drip out after sex? You are not alone in asking this common question. The semen does have a better chance of reaching inside the uterus and finding the egg when there is more seminal fluid enabling easier travel.

Don't panic, losing some semen is going to happen and it doesn't prevent conception. However, many women will take a pillow following intercourse and place it below the pelvis raising their hips about 3 to 4 inches. This is done to allow gravity to assist with drawing the seminal fluid towards the cervix opening and into the uterus.

However, there is no scientific data that confirms that raising your hips after ejaculation or standing on your head will improve your chances of conception. But it does seem like good common sense to raise your hips a little and let gravity help without going to extremes.

Frequency Of Sex

It is not so much how you do it – it's more important how often you do it. The frequency of sex directly impacts the quantity and quality of a man's sperm. If too frequent, then the sperm are immature and not as effective. If he goes over a week without ejaculation, then the fluid will be filled with a high number of dead or damaged sperm.

It is recommended that couples have sex every other day during the 14-day fertile phase of her cycle to maximize the health of the sperm available for fertilization. If you can't manage every other day, then try for at least every three days.

Timing Of Sex

Men are most fertile, and sperm is most plentiful in the morning after a good night's rest. It might make sense to switch to sex in the morning before you start your day. The important thing is to be flexible and prevent sex from being a chore. If you can switch to mornings, do so. Just make sure you keep your sex at regular intervals no matter what time of day it is.

What Not to Do

There are some things before, during and after sex that negatively affect your chances of conceiving and should be avoided.

- No hot tubs. Avoid hot tubs before sex because the high temperature can quickly kill off sperm.

- No douching before or after sex. Seems obvious but requires repeating. Douching alters the acidity of your vagina killing sperm and washing away the cervical mucus.

- No romantic baths. Again, the temperatures and soap can kill sperm

- No surfing on the laptop beforehand. The heat from a laptop placed near the groin is hot enough to kill sperm.

- Do not use lubricants that might contain spermicide. If you do need a lubricant, read the label carefully!

- No antihistamines (for women). Antihistamines are just as effective at drying up your cervical mucus as they are in drying up your nose. This will prevent sperm from reaching the uterus.

CHAPTER EIGHT

Conceiving At Old Age

Whether it is a later marriage in life, career paths or some other reason, the average age of couples starting families is getting older. Starting families at age 30 or older is becoming commonplace.

Although there are challenges that come with maturity and fertility, conceiving naturally is still possible for those even as old as 50. If you are in your late 30s or beyond, this chapter will provide you with insights on what challenges you may face and steps you can take to increase your chances of conceiving.

Challenges Of Conceiving After Age 35

As you start to age, your muscles and other systems in the body start to become less efficient than they were in your 20s. The same is true for the fertility of both you and your spouse. The egg quality as well as quantity both decline with age. It is also possible that you may be experiencing sporadic ovulation as you get older. Skipping or missing ovulation reduces your fertility probabilities by removing opportunities to even try and conceive.

There are also health conditions that impact your conception efforts or ability to carry a baby to term. Although these conditions may be experienced by younger women, the likelihood of their presence is greater with women who are getting into their 30s or 40s. Here is a list of conditions that may create a challenge for your efforts to conceive:

- Fibroids
- Endometriosis
- Less cervical fluid
- High blood pressure or diabetes
- Chromosomal abnormalities

If you have any of the above medical conditions, please consult your doctor before trying to conceive.

What Can You Do to Increase Your Chances of Conceiving?

Getting pregnant at ages 35 and older is more likely for women who are in better health. As noted, many times before, healthy conception is related to healthy you. Even if you have not made a habit of eating a healthy diet and exercising regularly, it is not too late to start.

Getting your body in the best shape it can be is one of the best ways you can invest in your fertility health. Where the average time for conception for women to conceive in their 20s is six months to a year, the average time for those in their 30s is between 1 to 2 years. Investing in your health all along the way is one of the best ways to increase your chances of conception.

Make sure that you are forgoing any lifestyle habits that can impede your ability to conceive. This means avoiding alcohol, nicotine, illicit drugs, and caffeine.

Be certain that you are getting the nutrients that you need including folic acid, calcium, and omega-3s. Zinc has been identified as a nutrient that is directly related to the fertility health of both you and your husband. In addition to eating well-balanced nutritional meals, you both can take vitamin supplements to make sure you are getting what you need.

Get Your Check-ups!

Because age is directly related to the fertility health of both you and your partner, you both must get a physical examination to make sure that things are working correctly. It is even more important for those over 35 because of the increased likelihood that you could be experiencing conditions like endometriosis.

Some conditions can be treated to bring your body right back to a viable state for conceiving. However, you may discover that conceiving is not possible. It is much better to know this upfront as opposed to experiencing months of stress and making unnecessary changes to your life.

Talk to your doctor – knowing what your body is doing is a big step for conceiving in your 40s.

CHAPTER NINE

Timing Intercourse for Gender Selection

Trying to influence the sex of your baby has been something couples have done for generations upon generations. A popular method for gender selection, the Shettles Method, was developed by Landrum B. Shettles in the 1960s and outlined in his book *How to Choose the Sex of Your Baby*.

Most methods for gender selection during conception rely on variations in the timing of intercourse, sexual position, and female orgasm. There are no guarantees and only observational data that suggest things you can do to increase your chances of one gender type over another.

Let us reiterate, there are no guarantees. You can read through the following suggestions for trying to conceive either a boy or a girl and judge for yourself.

Key Insights for Having a Boy:

Both the Shettles Method and Toni Weschler, author of *Taking Charge of Your Fertility*, make the following suggestions for trying to have a boy:

1. Male sperm tend to be faster, so having sex closer to the day of ovulation increases the probability that one of

the faster male sperm reaches the egg before the heavier and slower female sperm.

2. Artificial Insemination favours having a boy because the procedure is done closer to ovulation

3. Younger men and women seem more likely to have male babies. The hypothesis here is that younger couples have higher sperm counts and favourable cervical fluid which is an advantage to the male sperm

4. Based on fertility awareness practices, intercourse should be timed for the peak day and the day after, to increase the chances of having a boy. If you are using ovulation tests, you should test two times a day and have sex 12 to 24 hours after an LH surge

Key Insights for Having a Girl:
Weschler adds these suggestions to increase your chances of having a girl:

1. Low sperm count tends to favour the female sperm because they tend to be heartier.

2. Men exposed to hazardous chemicals, unhealthy environments, or other activities that cause the testicles to overheat are more likely to have girls. Again, the reason is believed to be that the female sperm are heartier and survive some of the activities that destroy the male sperm.

3. Where the *artificial insemination* procedure favours boys, the *in vitro fertilization* procedure favours girls.

The hypothesis behind this observation is again related to the idea of the female sperm being heartier and surviving the stress of the IVF extraction and procedure.

4. Based on fertility awareness practices, intercourse should be timed 2 to 4 days before your Peak Day. The female sperm are the ones more likely to live 3 to 5 days giving you a better chance of having a girl.

As a reminder, there are no guarantees no matter what you try. Scientific studies have failed to show a correlation between these techniques and the resulting gender of the baby. With that in mind, you may want to ask yourself which do you want more – a boy or a girl? Or is it more important to have a baby no matter the sex?

If you are focused on having either a girl or a boy, you are limiting your conception efforts and therefore significantly lowering your chances of conception each month. That is an important factor you should consider before trying to influence the sex of your baby with no guarantee of success.

CHAPTER TEN

Symptoms of Pregnancy

Now that we have discussed in detail all the possible things you can do to help enhance your fertility and get pregnant naturally, it's time that you learn to recognize the early signs and symptoms of pregnancy should you get pregnant in the future. Recognizing these symptoms is important because pregnancy symptoms differ from woman to woman and pregnancy to pregnancy.

Moreover, if you have no idea of any signs of pregnancy, you might mistake a common symptom for something else. For example, fatigue related to pregnancy might be brushed off as random stress and will not be taken seriously. Therefore, you might not make the extra effort to do something about it.

Another reason why understanding the signs and symptoms of pregnancy is important is because each symptom may be related to something other than pregnancy and could be a serious illness.

How Would You Know You Are Pregnant?

Some women experience the signs and symptoms of pregnancy within the first week of conception. For others, symptoms develop only after a few weeks or may not be present at all.

Below is a list of some of the most common pregnancy signs and symptoms. Some of these symptoms are considered the very early signs of pregnancy.

1. Implantation Bleeding

One of the earliest symptoms of pregnancy is implantation bleeding. This happens about 6 to 12 days after conception when the embryo implants itself into the uterine wall. When this happens, some women will experience spotting and cramping. *Other reasons for bleeding other than pregnancy are actual menstruation, altered menstruation, switching of birth control pills, infection, or abrasion from intercourse.*

2. Missed or Delayed Menstruation

This is the most common pregnancy symptom and when this is observed, a lot of women usually head directly for a pregnancy test. When you get pregnant, you will miss your next period. Some women still bleed while being pregnant, but the bleeding is shorter or lesser than normal. *Other reasons for missing a period other than pregnancy are stress, a certain illness, a food reaction, or a hormonal imbalance.*

3. Morning Sickness and Nausea

This is another well-known symptom of pregnancy that often manifests between 2 - 8 weeks after conception. You will feel nauseous throughout most of the duration of your pregnancy. Some women, however, are fortunate enough not to have to deal with morning sickness at all. *Other reasons for morning sickness and nausea other than pregnancy are food poisoning, stress, or other stomach disorders.*

4. Breast Enlargement and Tenderness

This symptom begins as early as the first or second week after conception. You may notice certain changes in your breast such as feeling soft and tender when touched, sore or swollen. *Other reasons for breast enlargement and tenderness other than pregnancy are hormonal imbalance, intake of birth control pills, approaching period (PMS).*

5. Fatigue and Tiredness

Tiredness, fatigue, and exhaustion are also signs of pregnancy during the first week. This is attributed to the changes in hormone levels as a result of conception. However, these will disappear once your body gets accustomed to the changes. *Other reasons for fatigue and tiredness other than pregnancy are stress, exhaustion, depression, common cold or flu or other illnesses that can leave you feeling fatigued or tired.*

6. Headaches

Headache is also the result of the sudden rise of hormones in your body. *Other reasons for headaches other than pregnancy are dehydration, caffeine withdrawal, PMS, eye strain or other ailments.*

7. Frequent Urination

This occurs around 6 to 8 weeks after conception. *Other reasons for frequent urination other than pregnancy are Urinary Tract Infection (UTI), diabetes, increase in liquid intake or excessive diuretics.*

8. Darkening of Areolas

The skin around your nipples darkens if you are pregnant. *Other reasons for the darkening of areolas other than pregnancy are a hormonal imbalance not related to pregnancy or maybe a leftover effect from a previous pregnancy.*

9. Food Cravings

Many women feel cravings for certain foods when they are pregnant, and this symptom can last throughout your pregnancy. *Other reasons for food cravings other than pregnancy are poor diet, lack of certain nutrients, stress, depression, or PMS.*

If you have been trying to get pregnant and are a sexually active person experiencing most, if not all, of these symptoms, start crossing your fingers because a baby may be on its way!

Good luck!

Disclaimer And Terms Of Use

The information contained in this book is for educational and informational purposes only. The content is not presented by a professional; therefore, the information in this book should not be considered a substitute for professional advice. Always seek the advice of someone qualified in this field for any questions you may have.

The author and publisher of this book have used their best efforts in preparing it. The author and publisher make no representation or warranties with respect to the accuracy, applicability, fitness, or completeness of the contents of the book. The information contained herein is strictly for educational and informational purposes.

The author and publisher disclaim any warranties (express or implied). The author and publisher shall in no event be held liable to any party for any direct, indirect, punitive, special, incidental, or other consequential damages arising directly or indirectly from any use of this material, which is provided "as is", and without warranties.

As always, the advice of a competent medical professional should be sought where necessary.